TEA WITH T

Let's Talk About Age Management, Eyes, Part 1

M. Theresa Turla, MD

To my husband, Pat: Your ever present support and patience drive me to continually explore my creative side.

CONTENTS

FOREWORD

Some say "the eyes are the windows to the soul." Nothing beats gazing into the eyes of the ones you love. But to many, the eyes are a mystery—the anatomy, the structures and the functions of each structure. Even physicians, who are not ophthalmologists, know little about the eye. They defer even the simplest ocular disorders to people like me, a professional ophthalmologist.

As an ophthalmologist, we are in a position to see all the age-related changes that occur with the eye. Many patients do not see an eye care professional until they notice changes in their vision and their eye appearance—usually seeing their eye doctor during their fifth decade (40 years old +) when they start having difficulty seeing up close or when they start noticing the wrinkles that surround the eyes.

The purpose of this book is to understand the mystery of the eye and to teach the reader how aging influences your appearance surrounding the eyes, how aging influences your vision, and how aging affects your eye health. But who wants to read a science book? You are curious but do not want to spend the mental energy to "figure it all out." Well, this book is for you. I should be able to explain any of these concepts easily over a cup of tea. And that is my goal for writing this book.

I tried to keep it as simple as possible to help you understand the basic principles of conditions and treatment. This book does not replace the advice you would receive from your own eyecare professional. It serves as an introduction so you can arm yourself with knowledge and ask worthwhile questions when you see the ophthalmologist.

"The eyes are the windows to the soul" is a romantic notion, but it also states a practical truth, "the eyes are the window to your health." We can diagnose high blood pressure, potential for a possible cerebral ischemia (stroke), diabetes, autoimmune disorders etc. Many of these conditions and many other age-related ocular conditions are not mentioned in this book due to limitations I imposed upon myself to keep this introduction to the aging eye as simple as possible. It's up to you, the reader, to let me know if you'd like a follow-up book that dives deeper into this subject of eye health.

Happy reading!

-M. Theresa Turla, M.D.

AT THE PLAYGROUND

Teagan saw Dr. Grace Foley all the time at the Metairie playground. Their sons are the same age, so Teagan often saw Dr. Grace at most of their sons' games. Throughout the season from football to soccer to baseball; and year after year, she watched Dr. Grace arrive, usually in scrubs and always friendly. Funny thing though, as the years passed all the other moms started to get face wrinkles, gain weight and complain of anxiety and mood swings; all the while, Dr. Grace did not. While all the other moms around Teagan aged, this one woman did not seem to gain a single wrinkle on her face, her skin remained smooth and bright, she kept her "girlish figure," and she was always in a cheerful mood. How does she do it? Then Teagan remembered a conversation from many years ago:

"As an ophthalmologist, I perform the usual… cataract surgeries and general medical eyecare," she said, "but I also give Botox, do chemical peels and fractional CO2 resurfacing. I also perform eyelid and brow surgery and I practice anti-aging medicine, otherwise called Age Management Medicine."

"I would never get Botox!" Teagan retorted. Back then, Teagan was in her early thirties and very beautiful. "I'm not judging, I just know it's a toxin and I don't want it in my body." Teagan looked at Dr. Grace cautiously as she expected her to argue in return.

"Meh," Dr. Grace shrugged, "No worries. T, I'll just see you in a few years."

Apparently, Dr. Grace was right.

WHY SO ANGRY?

Botox and Fillers

Teagan just turned 40 and she started noticing a few worrisome things. The most obvious is her wrinkles. She used to like the ones outside her eyes. Those lines proved to herself and to others that she smiled a lot. She liked these 'laugh lines' because it meant she enjoyed life and that she laughed often! However, recently, she noticed that they were getting deeper and remained on her face even when she was not smiling. With the addition of her skin losing its glow, these laugh lines were aging her. To top it off, her teenage daughter told her she had RBF and her daughter's friends actually avoided her, telling her, "Your mom always seems to be in a bad mood."

"What's RBF?" Teagan asked her daughter, Scout.

"It means Resting Bitch Face," she responded, "you look mad all the time, even when you're in a good mood. I think it's the wrinkles between your eyes, Mom."

Teagan frowned, then caught herself thinking, "Dang, that's exactly what's causing my RBF!"

She ran to the mirror and realized the permanent lines had developed between her brows that made her look angry all the time. She wasn't frowning at that moment, but it sure looked like it!

The next time Teagan saw Dr. Grace at the high school football game, she approached her and asked about these wrinkles in particular.

"Hi, Dr. Foley," Teagan said," how are you doing today?"

"I'm doing great! And please call me Grace or if you prefer Dr. Grace, outside the office! I just finished up my afternoon clinic and being here in this beautiful weather makes me so happy," she replied. "How are you doing?"

"Ugh," Teagan responded, "my daughter just told me I have RBF!"

Dr. Grace laughed, "Great acronym, huh? Resting Bitch Face. You would benefit from the use of

Botox, but I remember you said you would never do it."

"I hate that everyone thinks I am always mad when I'm not!" Teagan said, "but, I'm afraid of Botox. A little scared of the needles, but more scared about the poison."

"Well, one of the other moms we know comes to me all the time for Botox, and she loves it. You can speak to her if you'd like. She told me I can always use her as a reference, so there is no HIPAA violation."

"Yeah, I'm not really sure I am ready to get Botox yet. What's the worse complication you can get?"

"I like to say the worse thing associated with Botox is that you'd love it so much, you can't stop getting it, and it's not cheap. But in the bigger pic-ture, it costs about the same as a cut and color from a good and popular hairdresser," Dr. Grace said. "On a more serious note, there are very few complica-tions and I haven't seen any personally. However, one that is pretty bothersome for the patient is the risk of getting a droopy lid. But it is easily treatable and usually does not last long."

"Okay, let me talk to that other mom about what she thinks."

◆ ◆ ◆

Teagan had no idea that Jamie got Botox. Teagan was surprised when Dr. Grace gave her Jamie's name. Jamie is one of her closest friends.

Teagan and Jamie talk daily on the phone and they usually have lunch together at least once a week. Why hadn't she told me, Teagan thought. Now that she is thinking about it, Teagan had noticed how much younger Jamie looks for her age. Jamie is 5 years older than Teagan, but she looked 5 years younger.

Teagan arrived early for her once a week lunch with Jamie. She ordered iced tea and her usual salad with dressing on the side. Jamie arrived wearing gym clothes and was glowing.

"Wow, you look great!" Teagan exclaimed, "where did you come from?"

"I just came from the gym. I hired a personal trainer and just started working on resistance training," Jamie responded.

"I've always known you as a runner. Why are you doing that?" asked Teagan, as she sipped on her tea.

"Dr. Grace told me that as we age, we lose muscle. She said to add resistance training or weight training to build muscle but, more importantly, to keep the muscle we have now. I think I like it more than running now!"

"Dr. Grace is an ophthalmologist. Why are you taking advice from her?"

"She also practices Age Management Medicine. Sometimes she calls it Anti-aging Medicine or Lifestyle Medicine. She does it to help her patients age gracefully and to live life to the fullest!"

"Speaking of aging gracefully," Teagan started," Dr. Grace just told me you get Botox! Why didn't you tell me?"

"I have been getting Botox for the last 10 years. I don't hide the fact I get Botox. But I know how much you said you would never get it. So, I never told you. Why? Are you considering it now?"

"Kind of. My daughter just told me I have RBF."

Laughing, Jamie said, "Wow, that's harsh!"

"I know, right?" Teagan responded, "Can you tell me more about Botox?"

"I know you're afraid of Botox because you've heard of botulism," Jamie explained, "Well, botulism happens when canned goods aren't canned properly or if the cans you buy from the store are cracked. You ingest the poison from the food and it gets in your system and causes paralysis to the organs of your body. So, when your gut is paralyzed you have difficulty swallowing and you get GI symptoms like nausea and vomiting. It can go into your entire system and paralyze the muscle for breathing, and that's how you would die. Usually, it's caught in time and it's treated with an anti-toxin.”

“That sounds scary!” Teagan responded.

“The Botox you get is the same toxin, but it's injected directly into the muscles around the eye.”

“Why and how does it work?”

“Botox paralyzes the muscle, so it no longer contracts.”

“I don't want to have paralyzed muscles!” Teagan exclaimed.

“Yes, you do!” Jamie responded,” When you frown or smile, the muscles around your eyes contract. The skin that overlies the muscles folds, and that's when you get wrinkles. With Botox, the paralysis means no contraction. No contraction means no skin folding. No skin folding means no wrinkles!"

Jamie continued, "Think of it this way. Your skin is like a piece of cloth. When you make any facial expression, like a frown, the piece of cloth folds, creating a crease in the cloth. The crease is like a wrinkle. After you've folded that piece of cloth so many times, the crease gets deeper and deeper and can become permanent. The crease remains on the cloth even if the cloth is not folded. If you keep the cloth flat, you can, over time, decrease the depth of the fold. The same happens with the skin. When you frown, you're constantly folding the skin to make a crease in the skin, a wrinkle.

Botox stops the action of the folding of skin by *stopping the contraction* of muscle that causes the skin to fold. After some time of no movement, the wrinkle softens, and since the skin is forgiving, the wrinkle can completely go away! The younger you are, the more likely you can make the wrinkle completely disappear."

"Well, I am not sure if I am young enough!" Teagan exclaimed.

"Botox will still work. It will at least soften the wrinkle. And if you keep treating the area before any movement, the wrinkle will completely go away!" Jamie added, "I am sure there are those who arrive way too late, and their wrinkles are not only deep but also wide, and Botox may not be of any benefit. That's why you need to consult with Dr.

Grace to see where you stand."

"Why does this happen as we get older? I have been smiling and frowning my whole life! Why now?" Teagan asked.

"She said there are three stages, and they come on to patients at different ages depending on ethnicity, sun exposures, the environment and genetics," Jamie responded. "The first stage happens when you're young. You smile and frown and the skin and tissue under your skin is full and fresh. The skin and tissue show no signs of aging, there's lots of collagen and the skin is very elastic. So, there are no lines created at all when you smile at that age. You're smiling and frowning with no lines showing.

"The second stage is when you're in your 20-30's. The skin and the tissue underneath are now aging. There is less collagen, the skin gets thinner and it looks dull. The skin, which usually sloughs off quickly, now turns over at a much slower pace and becomes less elastic. When you frown or smile at this age, the lines show up between your eyebrows and outside the corners of your eyes, respectively. But at rest, when you're not using the muscles to express yourself, the lines disappear.

"Finally, at the third stage, the overlying skin has lost so much tissue, collagen, and elasticity and has become so thin and less bright. The lines that you had been creating at the same area, year after year, moment after moments of joy and anger; those lines? They remain, long after you have smiled or frowned. Thus," she concluded," resulting in RBF—resting bitch face. You look angry even when your face is at rest."

Teagan was attentive the entire time Jamie spoke. She finally understood what she was talking about. "How about you? How come you don't have any of those lines at all? You're older than me. It can't be genetics or the sun. I know your mom and she looks older than my mom and your mom is younger? We both stay out of the sun. So why no wrinkles on your face? Why don't you have laugh lines or RBF?"

Jamie laughed, "Believe it or not, I have been seeing Dr. Grace for years! I started at the middle of the second stage. I was creating those wrinkles when I smiled or frowned but they were NOT there at rest. I did not want to have those lines at rest ever!"

"I notice that as you're talking, I still see expressions on your face. I've seen celebrities have frozen faces and they say it's from Botox, but you don't have a frozen looking face!"

"The so-called 'frozen face," Jamie said with her hand gesturing in air quotes, "is part myth and part truth. Some of those celebrities have had major plastic surgery that accounts for that frozen look. Rarely, it's due to Botox. Botox is better for the upper face and it depends on where you have the Botox and how much Botox you get. You should see Dr. Grace for a consultation. You can discuss your needs and fears and she will treat you accordingly."

"A consultation? What do you mean?"

"For a small fee, she will look at your overall face and advise you as to how to remain young looking. For the most part, women our age feel young, but when you look in the mirror, you're surprised with how old you look versus how young you feel! She will advise you as to the spectrum minimally invasive procedures and practices to major surgery. It all depends on you as an individual and what your specific needs are."

"What did she tell you? Whatever she's done for you has worked!"

"I not only get Botox, but I also get fillers. I used to have bags below my eyes that made me look tired all the time. She filled them with a filler and now I look refreshed! Also, I get filler around my mouth."

"Fillers?" Teagan said with a surprise, "I don't understand why anyone would need a filler!"

"As you age, you lose facial fat. Your face starts to look thinner. Throw in the loss of collagen and elasticity, I mentioned earlier, and all that combined cause you to look older. The analogy she uses is how a grape becomes a raisin!"

"I still don't get it," Teagan responded, as she took a sip of her cucumber-infused iced water.

"Well, today is actually a perfect day to talk about it!" Jamie said as she put down her salad fork. "I am actually due to get my filler done."

She pulled out a pocket mirror from her purse and she pointed to areas around her mouth. "See these lines that go from the outside bottom of my nose to the outside corner of my mouth? Those are called nasolabial folds. Then see the line here that goes from the outside corner of my lips straight down to my chin? Those are called marionette lines. Sort of like you would see on a string puppet doll.

"And finally, see these tiny short lines radiating away from my lips? Those are called smokers lines, but you don't have to be a smoker to have them. They are created when you sip from a straw, kiss or whistle. Your muscles contract to cause your lips to pucker and that's how those lines are formed. And just like the concept I mentioned about Botox —those lines aren't there when you're young. As you get older, your skin changes, and with repetitive movement, the lines will stay there permanently.

"All these lines are treated with filler." Jamie pulled out her phone, "Check out my picture here on my phone from seven months ago. See how I look just a little bit younger? That's because I had just had filler a few days before."

Teagan looked at the photo on Jamie's phone. Jamie was with her family and she almost looked like her children's older sister. Her face was not just bright but also smooth and the lines around her mouth were nearly gone.

"This is a lot to take in!" exclaimed Teagan.

"I know," Jamie said. "Pretty much, the main concept, Dr. Grace told me, is that when it comes to the face, depressions and elevations are what's noticeable. Smooth discolorations are not as noticeable and can easily be covered up with make-up. Botox and fillers are used to treat the depressions."

"What elevations are you talking about?"

"Pimples and moles. Usually, these are

treated when we are young, but some of us get adult acne. But that's another whole different story! Lucky for me and you, we don't have to worry about it."

"Yeah, but there's still a whole lot to digest!' Teagan said. The lunch was over, and soon, they had to pick up their kids at school. "Thanks so much for telling me all this. I just may try Botox!"

"Not a problem, T" Jamie said, "I will let you know when I see Dr. Grace again, and maybe you can join me to see how it all works."

"I would love that!" Teagan said. The women both stood up, grabbed their purses and gave each other hugs, planning to meet the same time next week.

Teagan saw Dr. Grace at the soccer field a few days later. She thanked her for referring her to Jamie to get more information. Pulling out her phone, she said, "here are a few notes I took, but first, let me find my reading glasses." She fumbled around her purse, looking for one of the many pairs of reading glasses she kept.

Dr. Grace smiled and said, "Have I ever told you about presbyopia?"

BOTOX AND FILLERS: SUMMARY AND ADDITIONAL INFORMATION

- Depressions on the face can indicate aging.

- Wrinkles around the eyes and mouth are a form of depressions (of the skin surface).

- The wrinkles around the eyes are typically

treated with Botox.

· The wrinkles around the mouth are typically treated with fillers.

Eyes and Upper Face:

° Contraction of the muscles around the
eyes create wrinkles.

° "Smile lines" or "crow's feet" are the lines
that radiate from outside your eyes to
the temples.

° "Frown lines" or "elevens" are the lines between your eyes. These are the primary

cause of RBF.

° Botox works by stopping the contractions temporarily (about 3 months), requiring retreatment.

° Before treatment, if the wrinkles are deep and constantly presents, complete removal of the depressions may require multiple treatments during several months or even over a year.

° It's imperative to get re-treatment before the muscles return to full function (contraction) to avoid the creation of the lines in the first place.

° **Potential side effects** *(this is not a complete list and others may occur. Please discuss with your doctor):*

- muscle weakness at the area and near the area where the medicine was injected–droopy lid(s)

- blurred vision, puffy eyelids, dry eyes, dropping eyebrows

- dry mouth

- headache tiredness

- bruising, bleeding, pain, redness, or swelling where the injection was given

- trouble swallowing for several months

after treatment, especially if treatment around mouth

– muscle stiffness, neck pain, pain in your arms or legs, especially if treatment used for headache

Mid-to-Lower Face and Around the Mouth:

° Aging causes the loss of facial fat and changes in facial bone structure.

° Both processes above are the primary cause of the aging process for the mid to lower face and around the mouth.

° Aging causes loss of elasticity and collagen under the skin's surface.

- The depression below the eyes are called "tear troughs."

- The depression from your nose to the outer corner of the lips are called "nasolabial folds."

- The depression from the outer corner of the lips down to the chin are called "marionette lines."

- Fillers replace the loss of facial volume of the mid-to-lower face and around the mouth.

° Fillers can last from 6-8 months, requiring re-treatment.

° **Potential side effects** *(this is not a complete list and others may occur. Please discuss with your doctor):*

– Signs of an allergic reaction, like rash; hives; itching; red, swollen, blistered, or peeling skin with or without fever; wheezing; tightness in the chest or throat; trouble breathing, swallowing, or talking; unusual hoarseness; or swelling of the mouth, face, lips, tongue, or throat

– severe irritation where filler injected

– severe swelling where filler injected

– severe bruising

– change in skin color (typically, bluish) at injection site

– Rare: severe and sometimes deadly side effects can occur when filler is injected into a blood vessel (you cannot see blood vessels deep in the tissue). Call your doctor right away if your skin turns white, if you have pain during or right after injections, or if you have a change in eyesight

– Rare: loss of eyesight and other eyesight changes can occur. Call your doctor right away if you have any change in eyesight

– Rare: stroke like weakness, confusion, trouble speaking or thinking, drooping on one side of the face, or change in balance. Call your doctor right away if these occur

Additional Information

1. Losing facial volume, elasticity and collagen

also contribute to the thinning of the lips, which also comes with age. This is treated with fillers as well.

2. You can treat the contractions around the lips with Botox, however the side effects are typically too severe and/or annoying for the patient. These include drooling, difficulty kissing, difficulty sucking (for example, with a straw) and difficulty speaking.

MY ARMS ARE NOT LONG ENOUGH!

Presbyopia

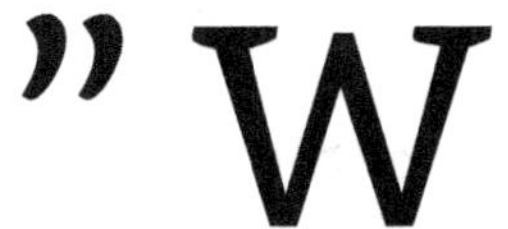

"What's presbyopia?" Teagan asked.

"Well, you probably never wore glasses until the last few years. Now you need them to see up close, am I right?" asked Dr. Grace.

"Yes! I had to keep pulling things away from my face in order to read! Soon, my arms weren't long enough!"

Dr. Grace laughed! 'That is such a common way to describe presbyopia."

"Well, I got quite a scare, so I went to an optometrist to see if there was anything wrong. Turns out I just needed glasses. She gave me a prescription for glasses to help for far and near, but I discovered that I only needed them to read. They were expensive too!

Dr. Grace listened and Teagan continued.

"I found out I can just use the over the counter readers I can buy at the drug store. Now I have them all over my house!" Teagan said suddenly," Wait, I just realized I have never seen you with glasses and we're the same age!"

"There are so many ways to treat presbyopia," answered Dr. Grace. "Let me send you to another friend of yours who can help you understand."

"Who is that?"

"Kim, the librarian at the public library."

◆ ◆ ◆

Both Dr. Grace and Teagan have been going to the library for most of their kids' lives. From storybook time when they were toddlers, to renting out Disney movies when their kids were tweens. In the past, Teagan had enjoyed holding a physical book as she read, often skipping the kindle/electronic book reader. Back then, who didn't love the smell of books and the absence of sound in a library? Kim, the always kind and helpful librarian there, was a common friend of theirs. Teagan often saw Kim with her grandchildren at the playground and at neighborhood picnics. Teagan thought back and realized that she never saw Kim wear glasses, although she was easily 20 years older than they were.

"I think I will go spend an afternoon at the library," Teagan thought.

◆ ◆ ◆

Teagan had heard that you can sign up for digital books at the library. She had not been there in years, ever since her children had outgrown "story-time" at the library. She decided to go there to sign up for a digital library card. While she loved reading physical books, she traveled often and liked to travel light. She used a kindle whenever she read on an airplane and on trips, choosing to carry-on luggage instead of checking in luggage.

As soon as she walked into the library, she immediately wondered why she did not go more often or why she had not been in years. The smell of the books is so distinct and immediately reminded her of the childhood of her children and her own childhood. The muffled silence comforted her and reminded her of the many years she spent studying within the 'stacks' of her college library. The staff greeted her with kindness and immediately offered help. She wandered through the library first, then approached the front desk.

"Can I help you," a young gentleman asked as she walked up.

"Yes, I am looking for Kim," Teagan responded. "Can you let her know that her friend, T, is here?"

"Of course, I will let her know. She is in the back office and should be here shortly."

"I can wait," Teagan responded.

Teagan waited and soon Kim arrived.

"Hi! So good to see you!" Kim exclaimed as she approached Teagan. "It's been a long time. I think the last time I've seen you here was when your kids used to go to story-time!"

Embarrassed, Teagan said, "Yes, I buy my

books off Amazon now, but I've forgotten how wonderful the library can be!"

"Yes, I love it here." Kim responded, "Is there anything I can do to help you?"

"I think you can help me," she responded, "Dr. Grace had referred me to you to ask about something called presby-something. And I wanted to ask you more about it."

Kim chuckled. "You mean presbyopia. Of course, I can share what I know about it, but it's not something that we can talk about standing here. I have a break in an hour. Let's meet at the cafe next door for some tea and we can talk then?"

"Wow, thanks so much! I'll just look around and borrow some books while I am here. I'll meet you over there then."

They agreed to meet later.

Teagan, meanwhile, finished up the application to borrow books online and found out that you can even download library books on the Kindle. Win! Win!

Soon, they met at the cafe, ordering tea and some scones.

After catching up on their lives and events, they soon got down to business.

"So, what can I do to help?" Kim asked.

"Well, I noticed that you do not wear glasses. Even though at this point in our lives, you should be wearing at least reading glasses, and you're not!

How is that?" answered Teagan.

"Well, actually, I've worn glasses my whole life, but I always wore contact lenses," she said. "When I turned sixty-one, I noticed I was having trouble driving at night from the incoming headlights. I saw Dr. Grace and she said that I had a cataract in both eyes. The treatment for cataracts is to surgically remove them, and then replace them with intra-ocular lenses."

"I am starting to have trouble with the incoming headlights at night too," Teagan said. "I can still drive, but every once in a while, they bother me and sometimes I have to look away. Especially new cars with the brighter headlights."

"Most cataracts start out that way. Until you no longer can tolerate it and you feel like you are in danger when you are driving at night is when you should get them treated."

"I see," responded Teagan. "It does not bother me that much, yet."

"The best thing about cataracts is that now you have an opportunity to get rid of your glasses. The intra-ocular lens they use to replace the hazy lens can be chosen just for you. Just like glasses or contact lenses, your eyes are measured for you specifically. The intra-ocular lenses are specifically chosen for you," Kim continued. "You can choose single vision lenses or you can choose what they call the premium lens so you could see far and near."

"I'm not really sure what a cataract is?" Teagan asked.

"Let's back up a bit. And talk about the lens of

a normal healthy young adult eye. Everyone is born with a lens that sits behind the colored part of the eye. You have blue eyes, mine are brown. Well, behind that colored part (called the iris), sits a lens. This lens is similar to the lens of a camera. When you try to take a photograph of an object at a distance, you need the camera lens to be zoomed out so you can focus on the object at far—say like the television at the end of a room. When you want to take a photograph of a flower in front of you, you zoom in, so you can focus at the near object. The lens inside the eye does something similar; for example, to read your text messages on your phone, the lens zooms in, by changing its shape, to focus at a near object—just like a camera.

When you are younger, the lens changes shape

easily when you need to see things up close. As you get older, the ability of the lens to change shape decreases. As the lens slowly loses its ability to change shape, it slowly loses its ability to focus up close. Therefore, as you age, you have difficulty seeing up close. Over time, the lens remains rigid and can no longer change shape. You then become completely dependent on reading glasses to see up close.

Teagan interrupted, "Can I recap what you just said? So, I can make sure I understand?"

Kim nodded in agreement and waited.

"So, the lens of my eye is like a camera lens. The relaxed lens in its normal shape gives me the ability to see far, but when I need to see up close, the lens changes shape so I can focus up close."

"Exactly!" Kim smiled.

"But… as I get older, the lens does not change shape so readily, and that's why I am having difficulty reading up close."

"You got it!" Kim said. "So that's when you pick up those reading glasses from the drug store, you are helping your own lens focus up close. If you wore glasses to begin with, like me, you would need to add the 'reader' lens unto your current eyeglass prescription, and that's when you start needing bifocals.

"Usually, you retain some ability to see up close, so the power of the reading glasses start out low, like +1.50. Then as you continue to get older, your eyes' lenses slowly lose all its ability to see up close; and that's why, at the end, you end up with lens powers at +2.50 or even +3.00."

Teagan said, "I find myself using the +1.50's pretty much all the time. But I have trouble keeping track of where my reading glasses are, so I buy a whole bunch and leave them all over the house, at work, in my purse and in my car. Good thing, you can get them at the Dollar Tree for just a dollar each."

Kim responded, "Yes, that is the problem for those who use only reading glasses—they lose them all the time because, for the most part, you don't need glasses to see! Only for up close! Good thing there are other options available. I tried these other options before I developed cataracts."

"What are the other options? "

"Contact lenses."

"Contact lenses?" Teagan inquired.

"Yes, there are two ways contact lenses can assist in the treatment of presbyopia. The first way is using one contact lens for near and using a second contact lens for far if you need glasses to see far. This is called monovision. The reason it is called monovision is because one eye is used to see objects at near and the other eye is used to see objects at far. Many people love this option but there are a few who cannot tolerate the difference between the eyes."

"So, since I can see far, I would only need one contact lens in one of my eyes to see up close?" Teagan asked.

"Yep. You can give it a try, that's what I did. But I didn't like it. So, I tried the second way."

"What's the second way?"

"The second way is using multifocal contact lenses. Each contact lens has correction for far and correction for near. Both eyes can, therefore, see far and near. Because of the profile of the lens, they can feel bulky and the lens can move around in the eye, so it would take getting used to it. Some people never get used to it. So, again, only a certain group of people can tolerate multifocal contact lenses."

"How did you do?"

"It took me like 2 weeks to get used to the lenses, but then I loved them! Dr. Grace said that to use either monovision contact lenses or multifocal contact lenses, you need to really hate wearing the reading glasses. Otherwise, you likely wouldn't do the work needed in order to get used to either method. She is right. I have a few friends that tried and ended up just using reading glasses or bifocal glasses."

"Thanks for the information. I'll make an appointment with Dr. Grace to see if I can give it a try." Teagan hesitated. "Hold up, what about your cataracts?"

Kim laughed, "I was wondering when you were going to bring that back up. I don't use contact lenses anymore because I have similar lenses **inside** my eye!"

"What? Really? What do you mean?"

"Remember, I mentioned the lens earlier that sits behind the colored part of the eye. Well, as we age, the lenses that we were born with become hazy. As a child, your lenses are clear. As you grow older, the lenses become opaque, sometimes turning yellow to brown, or sometimes turning to an opaque white. Your vision becomes cloudy due to the changes of the lens. Sometimes you can have severe glare with incoming headlights, even before your vision gets cloudy. They call this a cataract. They surgically remove the hazy lens and replace the lens with a clear artificial lens. The new lens placed in the eye is chosen specifically for you."

Teagan listened intently.

Kim continued. "What I mean is you could replace your biological lens with an artificial lens. The new lens is called an intra-ocular lens, because its 'intra' meaning 'in', and 'ocular', meaning 'eye'. Intra-ocular, in the eye. Normally, they try to cor-rect your eyes so you can see far with the new lenses. But then you would need to use reading glasses to see up close.

"But this is the time when you can choose your own lens. And just like contact lenses, there are two methods to try to avoid using reading glasses. And the concepts are the same as what I told you about the contact lenses:

"First, there is mono vision: one eye would get a lens for near, and the other eye would get a lens for far.

"Or second, both eyes can each get a multi-focal lens that has the ability to see near and far. Meaning, both eyes will be able to see far; and both eyes will be able to see near."

"Wow! So, they put the lens INSIDE the eye, instead of ON the eye?"

"Yes, whatever lens you and your doctor choose will be permanent. They will not change the lens out if you change your mind. So, you have to be sure. And there are advantages and disadvantages to each option. That's a whole other topic that I will leave to the professionals to explain to you."

"What lenses did you eventually choose?"

"This was an easy decision for me. Since I was already using multifocal contact lenses, I choose the multifocal intraocular lenses. It took me a while to get used to them, but now I love 'em!" Kim looked at her watch," Dang! My lunch break is up! I need to get back to work! You have my number, call me if you have any questions."

As Kim got up to leave, Teagan stood up and gave her a hug. "Thanks so much for your time and explaining things to me. That's a lot of information to digest!"

At the next high school pep rally, Teagan approached Dr. Grace.

"Thank you so much for sending me to see Kim. She gave me so much information on presbyopia. I already called your office to see if I have cataracts, and if I don't, I will likely try out contact lenses. I need to get rid of these reading glasses! They are so annoying!"

"Have you tried contact lenses in the past?"

Embarrassed, Teagan said, "Yes, I actually tried them out a few years ago. I was trying to have cat eyes for a Halloween costume and I ordered them online. They didn't work out too well. I wasted $100!"

Dr. Grace chuckled, "Oh, I see that all the time. You need proper education when first trying out contact lenses AND there's a huge risk of infection if you improperly handle them and if you keep them on your eye too long. What was the problem with you?"

"I could put them in and they didn't really bother me, but after about 30 minutes, I felt like I had two rocks in my eyes. They felt so dry!"

"Well, dry eye is also very common as we age," Dr. Grace responded.

"It is?"

"You have no idea," Dr. Grace said.

PRESBYOPIA: SUMMARY AND ADDITIONAL INFORMATION:

· We all are born with a lens that sits behind

the iris inside the eye.

· This lens starts out clear and flexible. It

can change its shape to focus at objects up

close.

· As you age, the lens loses its ability to see objects up close starting at the age of 40+. The usual and easy solution is to use over-the-counter reading glasses to focus at near objects.

· The lens looses its ability to focus up close gradually over time. You can typically start using over-the-counter reading glasses with the power +1.50. Initially, you may notice, on certain days, you do not need to use the reading glasses. It is perfectly safe to go wtihout reading glasses--unless you notice that, without them, you get headaches when performing visual tasks. Other days, you will notice you will need them. Over time, you will eventually become dependent on the glasses and will need to increase the power from +1.50 to +1.75 to +2.00 etc over time.

· If you desire to **not wear glasses**, there are two solutions:

-->Monovision *contact lenses,* or multifocal *contact lenses*

-->Monovision *intra-ocular lenses* , or multifocal *intra-ocular lenses*

Monovision:

- **<u>One eye</u>** is given correction (with contact lens or intra-ocular lens) to see objects up close. If you try to see an object at far with this eye, the object would appear blurred.

- **<u>The other eye</u>** is given correction (with contact lens or intra-ocular lens) to see objects far away. If you try to see an object up close with this eye, the object would appear blurred.

- *For contact lenses:*

- If you have not worn glasses for most of your life, usually, this means you will not get a contact lenses in distance-use eye. If you are myopic (near-sighted)/hyperopic (farsighted) and/or have astigmatism, you would receive the appropriate contact lens to see far.

- The dominant eye (see how to test for eye dominance in appendix I) is usually used to see far, however, this is not a hard and fast rule. Some people like to use their dominant eye to see near.

- If you already use mono vision contact lenses, you can opt to put in mono vision intra-ocular lenses, during cataract sur-

gery.

° If you have never used mono vision con-

tact lenses, you can opt to receive a trial

pair of mono vision contact lenses to use

prior to putting in mono vision intra-

ocular lenses, during cataract surgery.

Multifocal Lens:

·The lens is designed to have multiple focal

points in them, so you can see far and see near

with the same lens. You would need to put

them on (for contact lenses) or in (for intra-

ocular lenses) BOTH eyes. Therefore, both

eyes would see far and both eyes would see near.

·The science behind multifocal contact lens and multifocal intra-ocular lens are different and too complex for the scope of this book.

·The inherent design of these lenses can degrade the clarity of the image you see but is usually tolerable. In other words, you may be able to read the 20/20 line on the eye chart, but you may say "it appears fuzzy." The same goes with glare issues at night. When deciding to go with multifocal lenses, you need to decide how much wearing readers and or bifocals/trifocals bothers you vs how bothersome it is to have a less than optimal image, albeit minimal.

·Bifocal and trifocal eyeglasses are a type of multifocal lens where you train your eyes to look at one specific area of the lens for a specific distance: far, near, and intermediate (trifocal). "Progressive" eyeglasses have these properties with no dividing lines on lenses.

Additional Information:

For those who wear glasses to see far:

If you wear spectacles due to farsightedness (hyper-opia) or due to astigmatism, patients add a lens at the bottom of their spectacles. This is called bifocal spectacles, and patients use the bottom part of the lens to see up close. .

If you wear spectacles due to near-sightedness (myopia), some patients remove (or look above or below) their spectacle to see up close.

Some patients with myopia choose to use a bifocal to avoid the need to look above/below the eyeglasses or to avoid removing their eyeglasses, to see up close.

Regarding multifocal intra-ocular lenses:

1. Typically you can get multifocal intra-ocular lenses placed during cataract surgery. The

surgery will be covered by insurance, but the lenses will not be covered and you will need to pay the difference.

2. Some physicians offer these lenses to patients who do not have cataracts and wish to receive them. This surgery is then called a "clear lens exchange," since you are removing your clear lens (that has not become a cataract yet) and replacing it with a multifocal lens. The entire procedure is then considered an elective procedure (sort of like plastic surgery), and would not be covered by insurance. Please speak to your doctor prior to making this decision. Once the lens is placed in the eye, it cannot be removed (for the most part, it's

a complex decision made between the patient and the doctor). Also, you are replacing a perfectly healthy lens with a lens you are not used to, so you need to really really (I mean really) hate wearing glasses and contact lenses; enough to go through the risk and potential negative outcome of even a successful surgery, to go this route.

3. The scope of the advantages and disadvantages and potential complications of cataract surgery/clear leans exchange are too technical and advanced for this book. Please discuss with your eye surgeon.

A word on LASIK: Some choose to have monovision

LASIK. This is when the doctor surgically reshapes (corrects) the front surface of the eye (called the cornea) using a laser. One eye would be corrected to see close and the other eye would be corrected to see far. This is not common; however, some, who are very happy with monovision contact lens opt to have monovision LASIK. The scope of this information is too much for the contents of this book. Please discuss with your ophthalmologist.

WHEN I BLINK, I SEE BETTER!

Dry Eyes

At the pep rally, Teagan and Dr. Grace's discussion continued.

"I don't really understand what you mean," Teagan continued, "Of course, eyes can get dry. So, yes, 'dry eye.' Is that a medical condition? It sounds so simple like, 'wet hand' or 'cold feet!'"

"Yes, it's actually a medical diagnosis and is quite complex. Most people have a mild form and never see a doctor while others have it so bad, it can threaten their vision!" Dr. Grace continued, "There several causes and various types of treatments available "

"I do notice that as I got older, my eyes are more frequently red and when I travel to a dry environment, my eyes burn all the time." Teagan said, "I have traveled to the same places for years with no problem, but now when I go, my eyes are always burning and are red! I always wondered why. I would love to learn more."

"Okay, let me send you to another friend we have. I believe she's actually your neighbor. She had severe dry eyes and it took us some time to figure out how to manage her, but she is really happy now. It's Ms. Helen. She's little Angela's grandmother."

"Yes, she lives down the block and across the street from me. She has watched our boys in the past. I can easily give her a call."

"She's so happy that she said I can always use her as a referral. So, you should give her a call"

"I definitely will!"

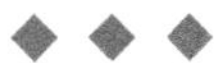

Teagan looked at the spread before her. She had the tea kettle on the stove and had baked shortbread cookies for Ms. Helen's visit. She had not seen Ms. Helen in a few months and was glad to be catching up on the latest family news and neighbor-hood gossip.

Ms. Helen arrived, all bright-eyed and smiling. They sat down for tea and spent much of the mid-morning talking and gossiping.

"Well," Teagan said when the conversation paused, "Can we talk about one of the big reasons I asked you over for tea?"

"Of course!" said Ms. Helen, "Dr. Grace had already called me to let me know you would be asking about Dry Eyes."

"Do you have Dry Eyes" Teagan asked. "Your eyes are not red and they do not look irritated at all."

"You should have seen me last year! Don't you remember that I used to wear sunglasses all the time. Even inside? I used to only like to see people outside so I can have an excuse to wear sunglasses. Now we are enjoying our tea indoors! What a treat!"

"Okay, so share with me what you know," asked Teagan.

"So, first, let me tell you that I am a retired nurse. I may get a bit on the technical side, so stop me if it's too much. Obviously, what I am about to say is a super simplified version of the science, but I will try to make it easy for you to understand."

Teagan nodded in agreement.

"Well, the obvious symptom of dry eye is exactly that...your eyes feel dry. They can burn, they can feel irritated and they can even make you feel like you have something in your eyes! Some contact lens wearers can no longer tolerate wearing their contact lenses. Some get glare, but sometimes the only symptom is blurred vision."

"Really?"

"Have you ever noticed that every once in a while, your vision can blur, but then it gets better when you blink?"

"Yes, that does happen to me every once in a while," answered Teagan.

"Well, that is just one of many symptoms of Dry Eyes. You can actually get blurred vision without your eyes feeling dry or irritated. Another crazy symptom for Dry Eye is tearing," added Ms. Helen.

"Yes! I've started tearing all the time when I'm outside on windy days! How can that mean that I have Dry Eyes?" ask Teagan, "It doesn't make sense!"

"Its actual a reflex, sort of like when the doctor taps your knees with a hammer. Your lower leg pops up!" Ms. Helen continued, "When your eyes sense dryness, you reflexively make more tears-- causing excessive tearing. It's counterintuitive but that explains it."

"Why does Dry Eye even happen in the first place," Teagan inquired. "We live in a humid environment.

"Because as you get older, you get dryer. Notice your skin, how it's gotten dryer? I used to never use lotion for my skin and now I use lotion all the time. The same goes for the eyes. Our eyes get drier as we age as well."

Teagan sighed, "Another thing we have to battle as we age…"

Ms. Helen nodded in agreement, "There are

tears that bathe your eye and its actually pretty complex. It's made up of three layers: mucous layer, aqueous, or water, layer and lipid, or fatty, layer. The decreased amount of the last two layers I mentioned are the main culprits for the cause of dry eye. The aqueous layer is pretty self-explanatory: less water means more dry."

Teagan followed along

"The lipid layer can also be decreased. It sits on top of the aqueous layer and when there is less lipid, the aqueous layer evaporates faster, then less water means more dry."

"That makes sense," Teagan said.

"That's one concept. Another one is about treatment. You can treat dry eye by several ways. First, is increase the amount of total tears/fluid on the eye. Second is decrease the outflow of tears/fluid that leaves the eye."

Ms. Helen continued, "The analogy I like to use is a bathtub that has two drains. Say you need to keep the same amount of water at the bottom of a bathtub, but now there is not enough water. You can turn the faucet up or you can put in a bucket of water every now and then to keep the water at a certain level. In other words, increase the inflow of fluid or tears.

"Another option is you can block one of the drains so the water already in the bathtub stays longer. In other words, decrease the outflow of fluid or tears." Ms. Helen added, "And lastly, you can maintain the health of the tear film—which I will talk about later."

"So, when my eyes are red, I use Vision or Murine. There are tons of tv commercials out there that say it's how you treat dry eyes."

"It's not suggested to use those drops for long term. If you use them all the time, once you're off of them, your eyes become even redder. It's called 'rebound' redness. If you have to absolutely have white eyes, say for a wedding or a job interview, that's when those drops can be beneficial. They treat the redness but not the problem."

"So, what should I use?"

"Well, to increase the inflow, you can use over-the-counter artificial tears," she continued, "you can take over-the-counter supplements that have omega 3's and 6's, and there are prescription medications. The pills you take increases the flow of tears and can take up to one to two months for you to notice an effect." She paused. "To decrease the outflow of tears, avoid dehydration. You can avoid fans, like overhead fans or fans in the car that point to your face. Point the fan away or use the fans that blow unto your feet. If you live in a dry environment, you may even want to consider using a humidifier in the room."

"Wow, I never thought of that. I do notice my eyes burning when I watch TV with the fan on," Teagan replied.

"Then the doctor can do a procedure to block the outflow of tears from your eyes using what's called 'punctual plugs.' We all have these two drainage holes in the inner corner of the lid, right next to the eye," Ms. Helen said, pointing to the area, "we have two them; one in the upper lid and the other in the lower lid. The doctor can place a plug in one of the holes of both eyes so the tears you naturally make stay around longer!"

"Sounds like there is a lot you can do to help with Dry Eye," Teagan added. "What do you do?"

"Well, my condition is a bit more complex. Remember I told you about the lipid layer of the tear film."

Teagan nodded.

"Mine was unhealthy. The source for this lipid layer are these tiny pores right on the lid edge, you know the area where some women put eye-liner? The area between the lashes and the eyeball? That's where the lipid comes from. It should come out like oil droplets but mine was coming out more like toothpaste. So, I didn't have a good lipid layer. I have to clean my lids—what they call lid hygiene. And sometimes I need to take a prescription pill to treat the secretions and make them more liquid-like."

Ms. Helen summarized, "So I do that; meaning, I keep my eyelid margins clean, take the prescription pill during flare-ups, I avoid fans, and I use an over-the-counter artificial tear that's specific to the lipid layers. With this regimen, I've been able to control my Dry Eyes!"

"This has been such an informative tea time! So much information to digest. Thank you so much for sharing!" Teagan stood up to give Ms. Helen a hug goodbye.

"Let me know if you need to know more," Ms.

Helen hugged back, "I'm just down the street." She gathered her things and waved goodbye from the front door.

Teagan stood alone, digesting the new information. "I'm looking forward to that appointment with Dr. Grace," thought Teagan.

DRY EYES: SUMMARY AND ADDITIONAL INFORMATION:

Typical Symptoms of Dry Eyes:

- Burning

- Dryness

- Irritation

- Foreign body sensation

- Blurred or double vision that goes away with blink

- Blurred vision

- Glare

- Tearing

The three layers of the tear film:

- Mucous layer

- Aqueous layer

- Lipid layer

Various Treatment options:

- **Topical (drops placed on eye)**

    - **NON-PRESCRIPTION DROPS**

        - Over-the-counter artificial tears with preservatives:

            >Evaporative (treats the lipid layer)

            >Non-evaporative (treats the aqueous layer)

Types: liquid, liquid-gel, ointment

>A combination of the above

• Over-the-counter artificial tears without preservative—if planning to use more than 4 times/day

>Individual containers must be thrown away if touch opening and/or opened greater than 24 hours ago

• Any over-the-counter allergy drop (allergies can give your eyes similar symptoms as dry eye)

- **PRESCRIPTION DROPS**

–Tear producing: Restasis or Xidra or Cequa

–Sometimes prescribed mild steroid drop but not for chronic use

–Sometimes prescribed antibiotic drop
—if concurrent corneal changes associated with dry eye

- **Medicines taken by mouth (pill)**

  –Omega's— flaxseed, fish oils—increase
  the production of tears (for example,
  TheraTears Nutrition supplement)

  –Doxycycline or similar classification of
  drug (prescription only)—to treat the
  lipid layer of the tear film (warning—
  avoid sun exposure and can cause GI
  upset)

- **Habits and new behavior:**

  –Avoid fans (overhead fans, car fans)

  –If using a nighttime CPAP machine—
  consider using nasal cannula and/or using

viscous lubricant (liquid-gel or oint-ment) prior to bed

–Lid hygiene (see appendix on how to make convenient at-home lid scrubs)

–Consider using humidifier

–Goggles when riding motorcycle, boat (anything that causes wind onto face/eyes)

- **Procedures that can be done in the office:**

–Punctual plugs—prevents outflow of tears from eye, keeping tears onto your eyes longer

–Expression of Meibomian glands in office

>>Manually—cotton tip applicators, expressing the glands at the slit lamp

>>With machine/technology (for example, IPL)—warms the lipid in the glands and removes the thickened lipid

T'S
CONSULTATION

"We finally get to see each other!' Dr. Grace exclaimed as she entered the examination room.

Teagan was a bit nervous. She had made an appointment to get Botox and to discuss options regarding her presbyopia (Teagan was actually quite proud that she learned how to say that word and actually know the definition!) and to potentially treat Dry Eyes.

Teagan has an aversion to needles, and the thought of needles injecting her face and even around her eyes made her nervous. She received her yearly flu shot and the occasional blood work required for her yearly exam, so using needles is no stranger to her. Typically, after each visit that required a shot or blood draw, she was always so pleasantly surprised that the pain did not match the anxiety.

"Hi, Dr. Grace," Teagan said nervously. "Ready to give me the shots?"

"Of course, this first visit is usually the longest visit because I need to make sure you understand exactly what is happening, the possible side effects, how long it lasts and so on. Did you answer the questions on our form? We just need to make sure you do not have any conditions that would prevent you from receiving the medicine. "

"Yes, I am pretty healthy. So, I think we can proceed," Teagan responded. Dr. Grace and Teagan then discussed when Teagan had learned about Botox through Jamie. After some time, Teagan asked, "Can I ask what is the most common problem YOU have personally seen with Botox?"

"Sometimes a small bruise can occur at the injection site. Rarely, your lid can droop, which typically goes away in a few weeks and can be treated with an eye drop. Luckily for me, this has never happened, but I have several colleagues who have experienced this. For the most part, the most common complaint is that you are going to like the out-come so much that you have to keep coming back! You may end up seeing me as often as you see your hairdresser!"

Teagan laughed at that. "Guilty as charged! I am not naturally this blonde!"

Dr. Grace smiled, "Are you ready?"

"As ready as I'll ever be," Teagan responded.

"Ok, here goes!"

After cleaning the areas with an alcohol wipe, Dr. Grace asked her to frown then relax. Then she injected the Botox between and above her eyebrows. Again, she asked her to frown then relax. Again, she injected above each eyebrow. Next, Dr. Grace asked Teagan to smile then relax. She proceeded to inject the outside area of her left eye. Similarly, she injected the outside area of her right eye. In less than a couple of minutes, the event was over. "Done! Keep your head elevated for the next hour or so. You will not notice the effect for 4-7 days, and it should last up to 3 months." Dr. Grace said.

"That's it? That was fast!"

"Yup! It sure was and it will be faster the next time. You'll already know what to expect." Dr. Grace continued, "We can now address your presbyopia. I already know you know what that is."

"Sure, I have been using over-the-counter reading glasses, but I find them annoying."

"Why don't we just give you a trial contact lens for your near eye and have you return in a month for a complete eye exam. If you like the contact lens, that's what we can prescribe to you. If you don't, we can try the multi-focal contact lens. Either way, the complete eye exam will let us know if you have cataracts or any other age-related eye conditions."

Teagan listened. She already knew what Dr. Grace was talking about.

"Finally, because of your occasional dry eye symptoms, let's start you on artificial tears and have you avoid fans. They do have artificial tears that you can place on the eye while you're wearing contact lenses—just check the label and make sure it says it's ok to wear with contact lenses."

"That's sounds like a good start. I will have to see how I feel with all these changes before I see you next," answered Teagan.

"Let me take you to my technician so he can

show you how to properly place the contact lens in your eye," Dr. Grace concluded. "He will let you know how to care for the lenses, as well."

As Dr Grace guided Teagan to the education room, Dr. Grace and Teagan hugged their goodbyes. "I'll see you at the next school function," they said in unison. They laughed and nodded, knowing there was so much more to be taught and to be learned.

APPENDICES

*Appendix I —Determining
Eye Dominance*

1. Extend your arms straight in front of you.

2. Open your hands, palms forward, forming a V between your pointing finger and thumb. Place hands next to each other so the V shape of each hand meet to create a triangle in the middle —thumbs overlapping at the bottom.

3. Keep both eyes open.

4. Look through this triangle opening at a distant object, like a doorknob or light switch.

5. Do not move your hands, arms, or head.

6. Close your right eye—do you still see the object? If yes, then you are left eye dominant. If you do not see the object, open your right eye then

7. Close your left eye—do you see the object? If yes, then you are right eye dominant.

Appendix II—Simple At-home Inexpensive Lid Scrub

You can buy over the counter lid scrubs made of wipes, or foam (for example, Ocusoft scrubs). Or you can create your own at home.

1. Get a foam dispenser—either buy a new one or you can use a pre-used one, such as Dial hand-wash foam dispenser. Just remove the liquid soap (and store for future use), clean the inside and rinse well, so there is no longer any Dial soap inside.

2. Place a small layer of baby shampoo, preferably Johnsons Baby Shampoo, at the bottom of the bottle.

3. Add water, fill to the top.

4. Gently flip the bottle upside down and right side up several times to dilute the mixture.

5. Press on foam pump.

What comes out is now a foam soap made of baby shampoo now safe to use on your eyelids. Remember to rub this foam at the base of the lashes, where the hair meets the skin of the eyelid.

Note: You can refill the bottle several times; however, every once in a while, replace the bottle with a new one to avoid mold/dirt build-up.

The End

About the Author:

M. Theresa Turla is a wife and mother who works as a locum tenens (traveling) ophthalmologist and has been in practice since 1996. She divides her time between New Orleans, LA, Charlotte, NC, and Roatan, Honduras. She values the patient-doctor relationship and strongly advocates the education of patients. She takes pride taking a complex subject and breaking it down to simple terms. In addition, she volunteers with Health in Sight Mission, an organization that perform surgeries for the indigent in Roatan, Honduras. When not fixing eyeballs, she enjoys travel, writing, scuba diving and snowboarding.

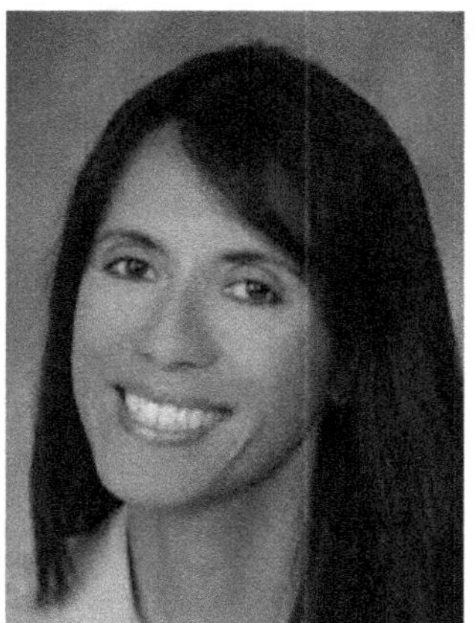

Photo by Steve Randon (using "photox")
Please click here to help me give the gift
of sight to the people of Honduras.